This Fitness Journal Belongs To :

Name : ....

Address: ....

Mobile: ....

E-mail: ....

DRIVEN RUNNER

Workouts That Target Specific Muscles (Front)

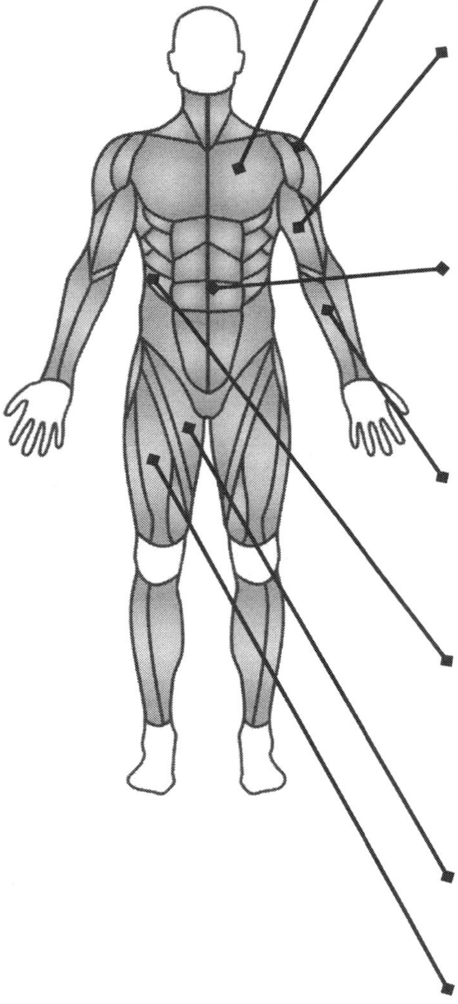

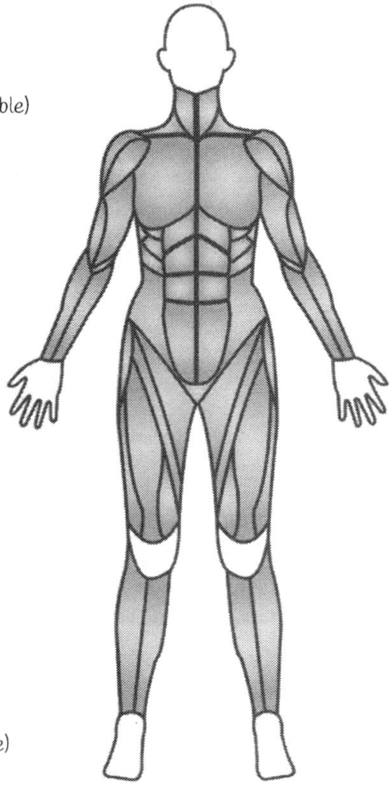

Chest
- Push Up / Press Up
- Bench Press (Dumbbell Or Barbell)
- Incline Or Decline Bench Press
- Weighted Push Up

Shoulders (Front & Lateral Delts)
- Shoulder Press (Dumbbell Or Barbell)
- Landmine Press
- Lateral Raise
- Front Raise

Biceps
- Chin Up
- Curtis (Dumbbell, Barbell Or Cable)
- Concentration Curl
- Drag Or Incline Curl
- Dumbbell Or Cable Row
- Underhand Lat Pulldown

Abs
- Plank
- Ab Rollout
- Captain's Chair Leg Raise
- Weighted Long Arm Crunch
- Leg Lift
- Leg Pull-in

Forearms (Grips)
- Two, Single Arm Hang
- Rack Pull
- Farmer Carry
- Dead Lift
- Wrist Curl And Extension

Obliques
- Russian Twist (Weightless)
- Torso Twist (Weightless)
- Wood Chop (Dumbbell Or Cable)
- Side Plank
- Side Bend
- Pallof Press (Cable)

Adductors
- Lateral Lunges
- Machine Adductors

Thighs
- Front And Back Squat
- Split Squat (Bulgarian Or Classic)
- Leg Extension Or Leg Press
- Step-up
- Lunge

Workouts That Target Specific Muscles (Back)

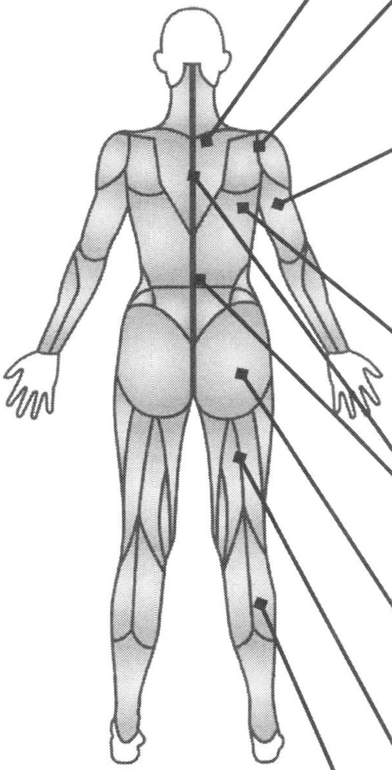

Upper Traps
- Shrug (Dumbbell, Barbell, Cable)
- High Pull
- Scapular Pull-up (Reverse Shrug)

Shoulder (Rear Delts)
- Bent-over Dumbbells Rear Delt Raise
- Dumbbell Or Cable Row
- Reverse Fly Or Reverse Pec Deck
- Face Pull
- Back T.Y & I Raise

Triceps
- Bench Press & Shoulder Press
- Close Grip Push-up Or Cable Push-down
- Overhead Tricep Extension
- Dumbbell Bench Press
- Push-up / Press-up
- Close-grip Push-up Or Cable Push-down

Lats
- Underhand / Overhand Lat Pulldown
- Pull-up
- Pullover

Mid & Low Back
- Row (Dumbbell, Barbell Or Cable)
- Rack Pull
- Back T, Y & I Raise
- Deadlift

Glutes
- Squat (Goblet, Barbell)
- Glute Bridge Or Hip Thrust
- Kettlebell Swing Or Pull Through
- Single-leg Deadlift

Hamstrings
- Romanian Deadlift
- Conventional Deadlift
- Sumo Deadlift
- Stability Ball Or Machine Hamstring Curl
- Glute-hamstring Raise

Calves
- Standing Calf Raise
- Seated Calf Raise

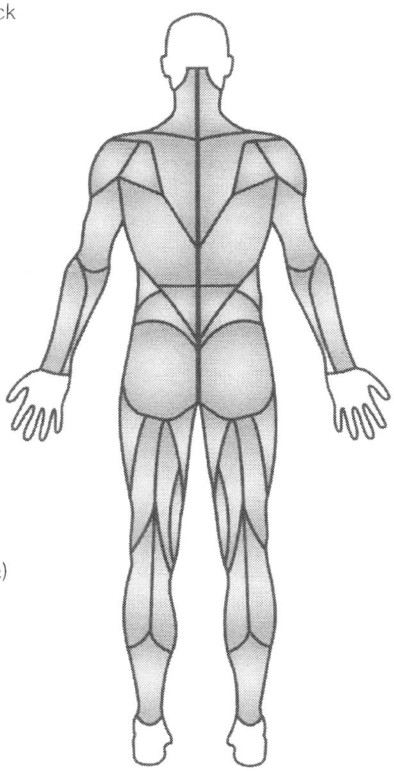

Calendar

C = CARDIO R = REST DAY W = WEIGHTS

MONTH:

SUN	MON	TUE	WED	THU	FRI	SAT

MONTH:

SUN	MON	TUE	WED	THU	FRI	SAT

MONTH:

SUN	MON	TUE	WED	THU	FRI	SAT

MONTH:

SUN	MON	TUE	WED	THU	FRI	SAT

MONTH:

SUN	MON	TUE	WED	THU	FRI	SAT

MONTH:

SUN	MON	TUE	WED	THU	FRI	SAT

Measurement Tracker

Week	Neck	Chest	Bicep	Waist	Hips	Thigh	Calf	Weight	Notes

My Starting Point

Date : / /

Weight

Body Fat %

Height

Before Front Image

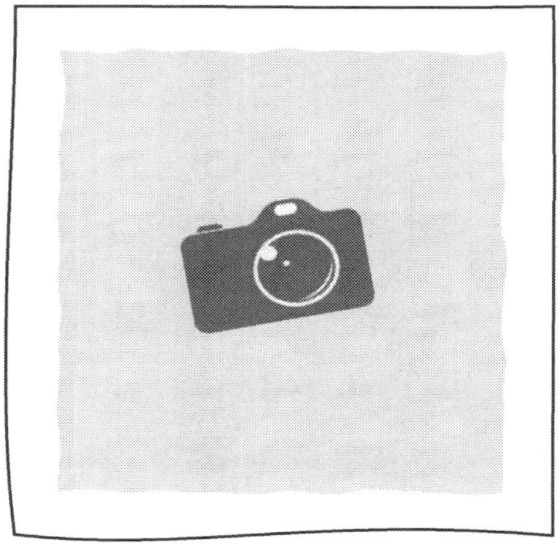

Before Side Image

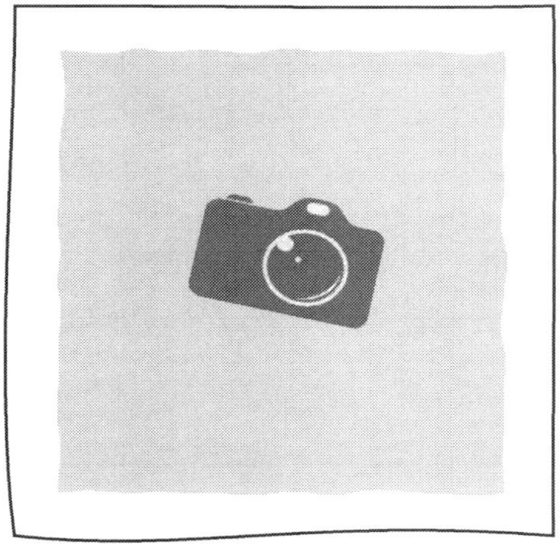

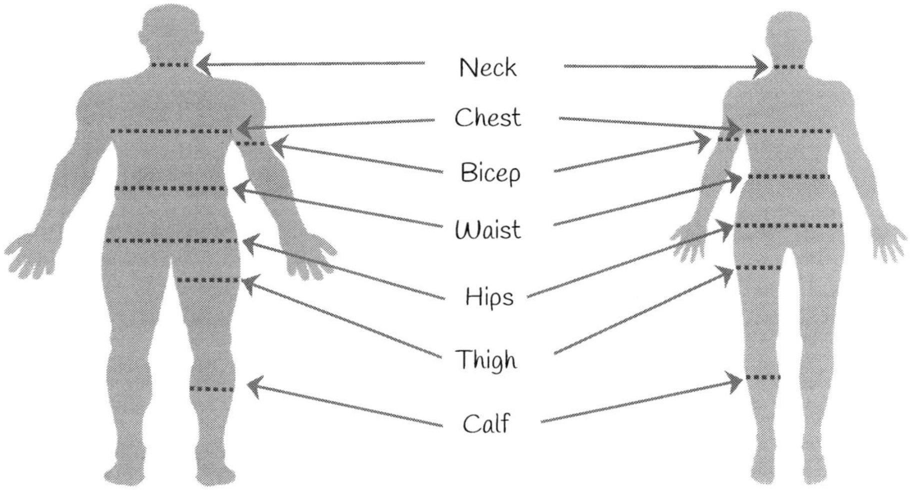

Current Measurements

Neck

Chest

Bicep

Waist

Hips

Thigh

Calf

My Goals

Goal #1

Plan

Deadline

Reward If Achieved

Goal #2

Plan

Deadline

Reward If Achieved

Goal #3

Plan

Deadline

Reward If Achieved

Goal #4

Plan

Deadline

Reward If Achieved

Goal #5

Plan

Deadline

Reward If Achieved

My Affirmation

Affirmations are a short powerful statement. It is the practice of positive thinking and self empowerment. when you say them or think them, they become the thoughts that shape your reality.

Date : / /

S M T W Th F S

How I Feel Today About My Food :

Today I Am Grateful For:

◇

◇

◇

Water :

Sleep Time :

Cravings / Response

Breakfast

Something To Make Tomorrow Better:

Lunch

Victory Of The Day:

Dinner

Notes

Snacks

Date : / / ☐ ☐ ☐ ☐ ☐ ☐ ☐ Weight Start

S M T W Th F S

Muscle Group Stretch ☐ Warm-up ☐ Finish

Affirmation

Cardio

Type	Time	Intensity/ Speed	Distance	Target Heart Rate	Actual Heart Rate	Cal. Burned

Exercise		Set 1	Set 2	Set 3	Set 4	Set 5	Set 6
	Reps						
	Weight						

How Did The Workout Go ?

Bad Ok Good Great

Date : / /

S M T W Th F S

Today I Am Grateful For:

Breakfast

Lunch

Dinner

Snacks

How I Feel Today About My Food :

Water :

Sleep Time :

Cravings / Response

Something To Make Tomorrow Better:

Victory Of The Day:

Notes

Date : / /

☐ ☐ ☐ ☐ ☐ ☐ ☐
S M T W Th F S

Weight

Start

Muscle Group

Stretch ☐ Warm-up ☐

Finish

Affirmation

Cardio

Type	Time	Intensity/ Speed	Distance	Target Heart Rate	Actual Heart Rate	Cal. Burned

Exercise

Exercise		Set 1	Set 2	Set 3	Set 4	Set 5	Set 6
	Reps						
	Weight						

How Did The Workout Go ?

Bad Ok Good Great

Date : / /

S M T W Th F S

Today I Am Grateful For:

◇

◇

◇

Breakfast

Lunch

Dinner

Snacks

How I Feel Today About My Food :

Water :

Sleep Time :

Cravings / Response

Something To Make Tomorrow Better:

Victory Of The Day:

Notes

Date : / /

S M T W Th F S

Weight

Start

Muscle Group

Stretch ☐ Warm-up ☐

Finish

Affirmation

Cardio

Type	Time	Intensity/ Speed	Distance	Target Heart Rate	Actual Heart Rate	Cal. Burned

Exercise		Set 1	Set 2	Set 3	Set 4	Set 5	Set 6
	Reps						
	Weight						

How Did The Workout Go ?

Bad | Ok | Good | Great

Date : / /

S M T W Th F S

Today I Am Grateful For:

◇

◇

◇

Breakfast

Lunch

Dinner

Snacks

How I Feel Today About My Food :

Water :

Sleep Time :

Cravings / Response

Something To Make Tomorrow Better:

Victory Of The Day:

Notes

Date : / / ☐ ☐ ☐ ☐ ☐ ☐ ☐
S M T W Th F S

Weight

Start

Muscle Group

Stretch ☐ Warm-up ☐

Finish

Affirmation

Cardio

Type	Time	Intensity/ Speed	Distance	Target Heart Rate	Actual Heart Rate	Cal. Burned

Exercise		Set 1	Set 2	Set 3	Set 4	Set 5	Set 6
	Reps						
	Weight						

How Did The Workout Go ?

Bad Ok Good Great

Date : / /

S M T W Th F S

Today I Am Grateful For:

◇

◇

◇

Breakfast

Lunch

Dinner

Snacks

How I Feel Today About My Food :

Water :

Sleep Time :

Cravings / Response

Something To Make Tomorrow Better:

Victory Of The Day:

Notes

Date : / / S M T W Th F S Weight Start

Muscle Group Stretch ☐ Warm-up ☐ Finish

Affirmation

Cardio

Type	Time	Intensity/ Speed	Distance	Target Heart Rate	Actual Heart Rate	Cal. Burned

Exercise		Set 1	Set 2	Set 3	Set 4	Set 5	Set 6
	Reps						
	Weight						

How Did The Workout Go ?

Bad Ok Good Great

Date : / /

S M T W Th F S

Today I Am Grateful For:

◇

◇

◇

Breakfast

Lunch

Dinner

Snacks

How I Feel Today About My Food :

Water :

Sleep Time :

Cravings / Response

Something To Make Tomorrow Better:

Victory Of The Day:

Notes

Date : / /

S M T W Th F S

Weight

Start

Muscle Group

Stretch ☐ Warm-up ☐

Finish

Affirmation

Cardio

Type	Time	Intensity/ Speed	Distance	Target Heart Rate	Actual Heart Rate	Cal. Burned

Exercise

Exercise		Set 1	Set 2	Set 3	Set 4	Set 5	Set 6
	Reps						
	Weight						

How Did The Workout Go ?

Bad Ok Good Great

Date : / /

S M T W Th F S

How I Feel Today About My Food :

Today I Am Grateful For:

◇

◇

◇

Water :

Sleep Time :

Cravings / Response

Breakfast

Something To Make Tomorrow Better:

Lunch

Victory Of The Day:

Dinner

Notes

Snacks

Date : / / S M T W Th F S Weight Start

Muscle Group Stretch Warm-up Finish

Affirmation

Cardio

Type	Time	Intensity/ Speed	Distance	Target Heart Rate	Actual Heart Rate	Cal. Burned

Exercise

		Set 1	Set 2	Set 3	Set 4	Set 5	Set 6
	Reps						
	Weight						

How Did The Workout Go ?

Bad Ok Good Great

Date : / /

S M T W Th F S

Today I Am Grateful For:

◇

◇

◇

Breakfast

Lunch

Dinner

Snacks

How I Feel Today About My Food :

Water :

Sleep Time :

Cravings / Response

Something To Make Tomorrow Better:

Victory Of The Day:

Notes

Date : / / S M T W Th F S Weight Start

Muscle Group Stretch ☐ Warm-up ☐ Finish

Affirmation

Cardio

Type	Time	Intensity/ Speed	Distance	Target Heart Rate	Actual Heart Rate	Cal. Burned

Exercise		Set 1	Set 2	Set 3	Set 4	Set 5	Set 6
	Reps						
	Weight						

How Did The Workout Go ?

Bad Ok Good Great

Date : / / S M T W Th F S

How I Feel Today About My Food :

Today I Am Grateful For:

◇

◇

◇

Water :

Sleep Time :

Cravings / Response

Breakfast

Something To Make Tomorrow Better:

Lunch

Victory Of The Day:

Dinner

Notes

Snacks

Date : / /

☐ ☐ ☐ ☐ ☐ ☐ ☐
S M T W Th F S

Weight

Start

Muscle Group

Stretch ☐ Warm-up ☐

Finish

Affirmation

Cardio

Type	Time	Intensity/ Speed	Distance	Target Heart Rate	Actual Heart Rate	Cal. Burned

Exercise

Exercise		Set 1	Set 2	Set 3	Set 4	Set 5	Set 6
	Reps						
	Weight						

How Did The Workout Go ?

Bad | Ok | Good | Great

Date : / / S M T W Th F S

Today I Am Grateful For:

◇

◇

◇

Breakfast

Lunch

Dinner

Snacks

How I Feel Today About My Food :

Water :

Sleep Time :

Cravings / Response

Something To Make Tomorrow Better:

Victory Of The Day:

Notes

Date : / / ☐ ☐ ☐ ☐ ☐ ☐ ☐ S M T W Th F S   Weight   Start

Muscle Group   Stretch ☐ Warm-up ☐   Finish

Affirmation

Cardio

Type	Time	Intensity/ Speed	Distance	Target Heart Rate	Actual Heart Rate	Cal. Burned

Exercise

		Set 1	Set 2	Set 3	Set 4	Set 5	Set 6
	Reps						
	Weight						

How Did The Workout Go ?

Bad   Ok   Good   Great

Date : / /

S M T W Th F S

Today I Am Grateful For:

◇

◇

◇

Breakfast

Lunch

Dinner

Snacks

How I Feel Today About My Food :

Water :

Sleep Time :

Cravings / Response

Something To Make Tomorrow Better:

Victory Of The Day:

Notes

Date : / /

☐ ☐ ☐ ☐ ☐ ☐ ☐
S M T W Th F S

Weight

Start

Muscle Group

Stretch ☐ Warm-up ☐

Finish

Affirmation

Cardio

Type	Time	Intensity/ Speed	Distance	Target Heart Rate	Actual Heart Rate	Cal. Burned

Exercise		Set 1	Set 2	Set 3	Set 4	Set 5	Set 6
	Reps						
	Weight						

How Did The Workout Go ?

Bad Ok Good Great

Date : / /

S M T W Th F S

Today I Am Grateful For:

◇

◇

◇

Breakfast

Lunch

Dinner

Snacks

How I Feel Today About My Food :

Water :

Sleep Time :

Cravings / Response

Something To Make Tomorrow Better:

Victory Of The Day:

Notes

Date : / /

☐ ☐ ☐ ☐ ☐ ☐ ☐
S M T W Th F S

Weight

Start

Muscle Group

Stretch ☐ Warm-up ☐

Finish

Affirmation

Cardio

Type	Time	Intensity/ Speed	Distance	Target Heart Rate	Actual Heart Rate	Cal. Burned

Exercise

		Set 1	Set 2	Set 3	Set 4	Set 5	Set 6
	Reps						
	Weight						

How Did The Workout Go ?

Bad Ok Good Great

Date : / /

S M T W Th F S

Today I Am Grateful For:

◇

◇

◇

Breakfast

Lunch

Dinner

Snacks

How I Feel Today About My Food :

Water :

Sleep Time :

Cravings / Response

Something To Make Tomorrow Better:

Victory Of The Day:

Notes

Date : / /

S M T W Th F S

Weight

Start

Muscle Group

Stretch ☐ Warm-up ☐

Finish

Affirmation

Cardio

Type	Time	Intensity/ Speed	Distance	Target Heart Rate	Actual Heart Rate	Cal. Burned

Exercise		Set 1	Set 2	Set 3	Set 4	Set 5	Set 6
	Reps						
	Weight						

How Did The Workout Go ?

Bad Ok Good Great

Date : / / S M T W Th F S

Today I Am Grateful For:

◇

◇

◇

Breakfast

Lunch

Dinner

Snacks

How I Feel Today About My Food :

Water :

Sleep Time :

Cravings / Response

Something To Make Tomorrow Better:

Victory Of The Day:

Notes

Date : / / ☐ ☐ ☐ ☐ ☐ ☐ ☐ S M T W Th F S Weight Start

Muscle Group Stretch ☐ Warm-up ☐ Finish

Affirmation

Cardio

Type	Time	Intensity/ Speed	Distance	Target Heart Rate	Actual Heart Rate	Cal. Burned

Exercise

		Set 1	Set 2	Set 3	Set 4	Set 5	Set 6
	Reps						
	Weight						

How Did The Workout Go ?

Bad Ok Good Great

Date : / / S M T W Th F S

Today I Am Grateful For:

◇

◇

◇

Breakfast

Lunch

Dinner

Snacks

How I Feel Today About My Food :

Water :

Sleep Time :

Cravings / Response

Something To Make Tomorrow Better:

Victory Of The Day:

Notes

Date : / / ☐ ☐ ☐ ☐ ☐ ☐ ☐ S M T W Th F S

Weight Start

Muscle Group

Stretch ☐ Warm-up ☐ Finish

Affirmation

Cardio

Type	Time	Intensity/ Speed	Distance	Target Heart Rate	Actual Heart Rate	Cal. Burned

Exercise		Set 1	Set 2	Set 3	Set 4	Set 5	Set 6
	Reps						
	Weight						

How Did The Workout Go ?

Bad Ok Good Great

Date : / /

S M T W Th F S

Today I Am Grateful For:

◇

◇

◇

How I Feel Today About My Food :

Water :

Sleep Time :

Cravings / Response

Something To Make Tomorrow Better:

Victory Of The Day:

Breakfast

Lunch

Dinner

Snacks

Notes

Date : / /
S M T W Th F S
Weight
Start
Muscle Group
Stretch ☐ Warm-up ☐
Finish

Affirmation

Cardio

Type	Time	Intensity/ Speed	Distance	Target Heart Rate	Actual Heart Rate	Cal. Burned

Exercise		Set 1	Set 2	Set 3	Set 4	Set 5	Set 6
	Reps						
	Weight						

How Did The Workout Go ?

Bad | Ok | Good | Great

Date : / /

S M T W Th F S

Today I Am Grateful For:

◇

◇

◇

Breakfast

Lunch

Dinner

Snacks

How I Feel Today About My Food :

Water :

Sleep Time :

Cravings / Response

Something To Make Tomorrow Better:

Victory Of The Day:

Notes

Date : / / ☐ S ☐ M ☐ T ☐ W ☐ Th ☐ F ☐ S Weight Start

Muscle Group Stretch ☐ Warm-up ☐ Finish

Affirmation

Cardio

Type	Time	Intensity/ Speed	Distance	Target Heart Rate	Actual Heart Rate	Cal. Burned

Exercise		Set 1	Set 2	Set 3	Set 4	Set 5	Set 6
	Reps						
	Weight						

How Did The Workout Go ?

Bad Ok Good Great

Date : / /

S M T W Th F S

Today I Am Grateful For:

◇

◇

◇

Breakfast

Lunch

Dinner

Snacks

How I Feel Today About My Food :

Water :

Sleep Time :

Cravings / Response

Something To Make Tomorrow Better:

Victory Of The Day:

Notes

Date : / / S M T W Th F S Weight Start

Muscle Group Stretch ☐ Warm-up ☐ Finish

Affirmation

Cardio

Type	Time	Intensity/ Speed	Distance	Target Heart Rate	Actual Heart Rate	Cal. Burned

Exercise

		Set 1	Set 2	Set 3	Set 4	Set 5	Set 6
	Reps						
	Weight						

How Did The Workout Go ?

Bad Ok Good Great

Date : / /

S M T W Th F S

How I Feel Today About My Food :

Today I Am Grateful For:

◇

◇

◇

Water :

Sleep Time :

Breakfast

Cravings / Response

Something To Make Tomorrow Better:

Lunch

Victory Of The Day:

Dinner

Notes

Snacks

Date : / / ☐ ☐ ☐ ☐ ☐ ☐ ☐ Weight Start
S M T W Th F S

Muscle Group Stretch ☐ Warm-up ☐ Finish

Affirmation

Cardio

Type	Time	Intensity/ Speed	Distance	Target Heart Rate	Actual Heart Rate	Cal. Burned

Exercise

		Set 1	Set 2	Set 3	Set 4	Set 5	Set 6
	Reps						
	Weight						

How Did The Workout Go ?

Bad Ok Good Great

Date : / /

S M T W Th F S

Today I Am Grateful For:

◇

◇

◇

Breakfast

Lunch

Dinner

Snacks

How I Feel Today About My Food :

Water :

Sleep Time :

Cravings / Response

Something To Make Tomorrow Better:

Victory Of The Day:

Notes

Date : / / S M T W Th F S

Weight

Start

Muscle Group

Stretch ☐ Warm-up ☐

Finish

Affirmation

Cardio

Type	Time	Intensity/ Speed	Distance	Target Heart Rate	Actual Heart Rate	Cal. Burned

Exercise		Set 1	Set 2	Set 3	Set 4	Set 5	Set 6
	Reps						
	Weight						

How Did The Workout Go ?

Bad Ok Good Great

Date : / / S M T W Th F S

Today I Am Grateful For:

◇

◇

◇

Breakfast

Lunch

Dinner

Snacks

How I Feel Today About My Food :

Water :

Sleep Time :

Cravings / Response

Something To Make Tomorrow Better:

Victory Of The Day:

Notes

Date : / /

S M T W Th F S

Weight

Start

Muscle Group

Stretch ☐ Warm-up ☐

Finish

Affirmation

Cardio

Type	Time	Intensity/ Speed	Distance	Target Heart Rate	Actual Heart Rate	Cal. Burned

Exercise

Exercise		Set 1	Set 2	Set 3	Set 4	Set 5	Set 6
	Reps						
	Weight						

How Did The Workout Go ?

Bad Ok Good Great

Date : / /

S M T W Th F S

Today I Am Grateful For:

◇

◇

◇

Breakfast

Lunch

Dinner

Snacks

How I Feel Today About My Food :

Water :

Sleep Time :

Cravings / Response

Something To Make Tomorrow Better:

Victory Of The Day:

Notes

Date : / / ☐ ☐ ☐ ☐ ☐ ☐ ☐ S M T W Th F S Weight Start

Muscle Group Stretch ☐ Warm-up ☐ Finish

Affirmation

Cardio

Type	Time	Intensity/ Speed	Distance	Target Heart Rate	Actual Heart Rate	Cal. Burned

Exercise		Set 1	Set 2	Set 3	Set 4	Set 5	Set 6
	Reps						
	Weight						

How Did The Workout Go ?

Bad Ok Good Great

Date : / /

S M T W Th F S

Today I Am Grateful For:

◇

◇

◇

Breakfast

Lunch

Dinner

Snacks

How I Feel Today About My Food :

Water :

Sleep Time :

Cravings / Response

Something To Make Tomorrow Better:

Victory Of The Day:

Notes

Date : / /

S	M	T	W	Th	F	S
☐	☐	☐	☐	☐	☐	☐

Weight

Start

Muscle Group

Stretch ☐ Warm-up ☐

Finish

Affirmation

Cardio

Type	Time	Intensity/ Speed	Distance	Target Heart Rate	Actual Heart Rate	Cal. Burned

Exercise		Set 1	Set 2	Set 3	Set 4	Set 5	Set 6
	Reps						
	Weight						

How Did The Workout Go ?

Bad Ok Good Great

Date :   /   /

S M T W Th F S

Today I Am Grateful For:

◇

◇

◇

Breakfast

Lunch

Dinner

Snacks

How I Feel Today About My Food :

Water :

Sleep Time :

Cravings / Response

Something To Make Tomorrow Better:

Victory Of The Day:

Notes

Date : / /

S M T W Th F S

Weight

Start

Muscle Group

Stretch ☐ Warm-up ☐

Finish

Affirmation

Cardio

Type	Time	Intensity/ Speed	Distance	Target Heart Rate	Actual Heart Rate	Cal. Burned

Exercise

		Set 1	Set 2	Set 3	Set 4	Set 5	Set 6
	Reps						
	Weight						

How Did The Workout Go ?

Bad | Ok | Good | Great

Date : / /

S M T W Th F S

Today I Am Grateful For:

◇

◇

◇

Breakfast

Lunch

Dinner

Snacks

How I Feel Today About My Food :

Water :

Sleep Time :

Cravings / Response

Something To Make Tomorrow Better:

Victory Of The Day:

Notes

Date : / /

S	M	T	W	Th	F	S
☐	☐	☐	☐	☐	☐	☐

Weight

Start

Muscle Group

Stretch ☐ Warm-up ☐

Finish

Affirmation

Cardio

Type	Time	Intensity/ Speed	Distance	Target Heart Rate	Actual Heart Rate	Cal. Burned

Exercise

Exercise		Set 1	Set 2	Set 3	Set 4	Set 5	Set 6
	Reps						
	Weight						

How Did The Workout Go ?

Bad | Ok | Good | Great

Date : / /

S M T W Th F S

How I Feel Today About My Food :

Today I Am Grateful For:

◇

◇

◇

Water :

Sleep Time :

Cravings / Response

Breakfast

Something To Make Tomorrow Better:

Lunch

Victory Of The Day:

Dinner

Notes

Snacks

Date : / /

S M T W Th F S

Weight

Start

Muscle Group

Stretch ☐ Warm-up ☐

Finish

Affirmation

Cardio

Type	Time	Intensity/ Speed	Distance	Target Heart Rate	Actual Heart Rate	Cal. Burned

Exercise

Exercise		Set 1	Set 2	Set 3	Set 4	Set 5	Set 6
	Reps						
	Weight						

How Did The Workout Go ?

Bad Ok Good Great

Date : / / S M T W Th F S

Today I Am Grateful For:

◇

◇

◇

Breakfast

Lunch

Dinner

Snacks

How I Feel Today About My Food :

Water :

Sleep Time :

Cravings / Response

Something To Make Tomorrow Better:

Victory Of The Day:

Notes

Date : / / ☐ ☐ ☐ ☐ ☐ ☐ ☐ S M T W Th F S Weight Start

Muscle Group Stretch ☐ Warm-up ☐ Finish

Affirmation

Cardio

Type	Time	Intensity/ Speed	Distance	Target Heart Rate	Actual Heart Rate	Cal. Burned

Exercise

Exercise		Set 1	Set 2	Set 3	Set 4	Set 5	Set 6
	Reps						
	Weight						

How Did The Workout Go ?

Bad Ok Good Great

Date : / /

S M T W Th F S

Today I Am Grateful For:

◇

◇

◇

Breakfast

Lunch

Dinner

Snacks

How I Feel Today About My Food :

Water :

Sleep Time :

Cravings / Response

Something To Make Tomorrow Better:

Victory Of The Day:

Notes

Date : / / S M T W Th F S Weight Start

Muscle Group Stretch Warm-up Finish

Affirmation

Cardio

Type	Time	Intensity/ Speed	Distance	Target Heart Rate	Actual Heart Rate	Cal. Burned

Exercise		Set 1	Set 2	Set 3	Set 4	Set 5	Set 6
	Reps						
	Weight						

How Did The Workout Go ?

Bad Ok Good Great

Date : / /

S M T W Th F S

Today I Am Grateful For:

◇

◇

◇

Breakfast

Lunch

Dinner

Snacks

How I Feel Today About My Food :

Water :

Sleep Time :

Cravings / Response

Something To Make Tomorrow Better:

Victory Of The Day:

Notes

Date : / /

S M T W Th F S

Weight

Start

Muscle Group

Stretch ☐ Warm-up ☐

Finish

Affirmation

Cardio

Type	Time	Intensity/ Speed	Distance	Target Heart Rate	Actual Heart Rate	Cal. Burned

Exercise		Set 1	Set 2	Set 3	Set 4	Set 5	Set 6
	Reps						
	Weight						

How Did The Workout Go ?

Bad Ok Good Great

Date :   /   /

S M T W Th F S

Today I Am Grateful For:

◇

◇

◇

Breakfast

Lunch

Dinner

Snacks

How I Feel Today About My Food :

Water :

Sleep Time :

Cravings / Response

Something To Make Tomorrow Better:

Victory Of The Day:

Notes

Date : / / ☐ S ☐ M ☐ T ☐ W ☐ Th ☐ F ☐ S Weight Start

Muscle Group Stretch ☐ Warm-up ☐ Finish

Affirmation

Cardio

Type	Time	Intensity/ Speed	Distance	Target Heart Rate	Actual Heart Rate	Cal. Burned

Exercise		Set 1	Set 2	Set 3	Set 4	Set 5	Set 6
	Reps						
	Weight						

How Did The Workout Go ?

☐ Bad ☐ Ok ☐ Good ☐ Great

Results

Date : / /

Weight

Body Fat %

Height

Front Image

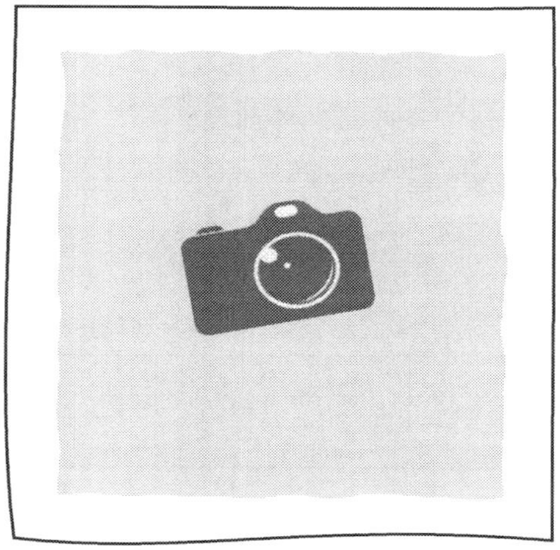

Side Image

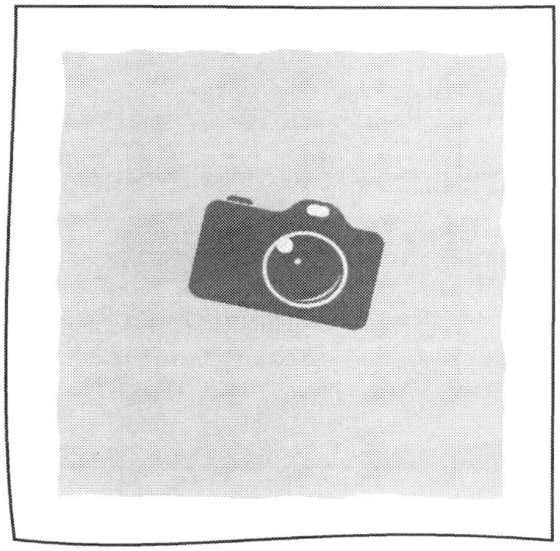

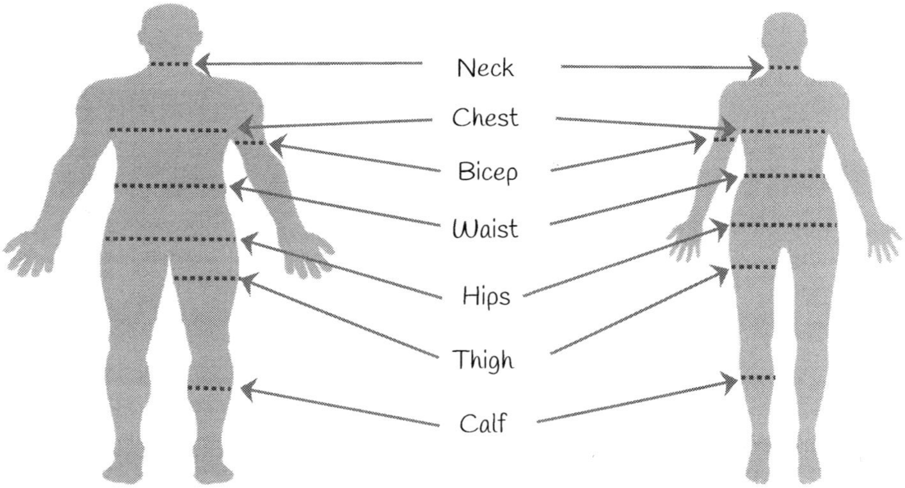

Measurements

Neck

Chest

Bicep

Waist

Hips

Thigh

Calf

My Goals

Goal #1

Plan

Deadline

Reward If Achieved

Goal #2

Plan

Deadline

Reward If Achieved

Goal #3

Plan

Deadline

Reward If Achieved

Goal #4

Plan

Deadline

Reward If Achieved

Goal #5

Plan

Deadline

Reward If Achieved

Notes

Date : / /

S M T W Th F S

Today I Am Grateful For:

◇

◇

◇

Breakfast

Lunch

Dinner

Snacks

How I Feel Today About My Food :

Water :

Sleep Time :

Cravings / Response

Something To Make Tomorrow Better:

Victory Of The Day:

Notes

Date : / / ☐ S ☐ M ☐ T ☐ W ☐ Th ☐ F ☐ S Weight Start

Muscle Group Stretch ☐ Warm-up ☐ Finish

Affirmation

Cardio

Type	Time	Intensity/ Speed	Distance	Target Heart Rate	Actual Heart Rate	Cal. Burned

Exercise		Set 1	Set 2	Set 3	Set 4	Set 5	Set 6
	Reps						
	Weight						

How Did The Workout Go ?

Bad Ok Good Great

Date : / /

S M T W Th F S

Today I Am Grateful For:

◇

◇

◇

Breakfast

Lunch

Dinner

Snacks

How I Feel Today About My Food :

Water :

Sleep Time :

Cravings / Response

Something To Make Tomorrow Better:

Victory Of The Day:

Notes

Date : / / ☐ ☐ ☐ ☐ ☐ ☐ ☐ Weight Start
S M T W Th F S

Muscle Group Stretch ☐ Warm-up ☐ Finish

Affirmation

Cardio

Type	Time	Intensity/ Speed	Distance	Target Heart Rate	Actual Heart Rate	Cal. Burned

Exercise

		Set 1	Set 2	Set 3	Set 4	Set 5	Set 6
	Reps						
	Weight						

How Did The Workout Go ?

Bad Ok Good Great

Date : / /

S M T W Th F S

Today I Am Grateful For:

◇

◇

◇

Breakfast

Lunch

Dinner

Snacks

How I Feel Today About My Food :

Water :

Sleep Time :

Cravings / Response

Something To Make Tomorrow Better:

Victory Of The Day:

Notes

Date : / / S M T W Th F S Weight Start

Muscle Group Stretch ☐ Warm-up ☐ Finish

Affirmation

Cardio

Type	Time	Intensity/ Speed	Distance	Target Heart Rate	Actual Heart Rate	Cal. Burned

Exercise		Set 1	Set 2	Set 3	Set 4	Set 5	Set 6
	Reps						
	Weight						

How Did The Workout Go ?

Bad Ok Good Great

Date : / / S M T W Th F S

Today I Am Grateful For:

◇

◇

◇

Breakfast

Lunch

Dinner

Snacks

How I Feel Today About My Food :

Water :

Sleep Time :

Cravings / Response

Something To Make Tomorrow Better:

Victory Of The Day:

Notes

Date : / / ☐ ☐ ☐ ☐ ☐ ☐ ☐
S M T W Th F S

Weight Start

Muscle Group

Stretch ☐ Warm-up ☐ Finish

Affirmation

Cardio

Type	Time	Intensity/ Speed	Distance	Target Heart Rate	Actual Heart Rate	Cal. Burned

Exercise		Set 1	Set 2	Set 3	Set 4	Set 5	Set 6
	Reps						
	Weight						

How Did The Workout Go ?

Bad Ok Good Great

Date : / /

S M T W Th F S

Today I Am Grateful For:

◇

◇

◇

Breakfast

Lunch

Dinner

Snacks

How I Feel Today About My Food :

Water :

Sleep Time :

Cravings / Response

Something To Make Tomorrow Better:

Victory Of The Day:

Notes

Date : / / S M T W Th F S Weight Start

Muscle Group Stretch ☐ Warm-up ☐ Finish

Affirmation

Cardio

Type	Time	Intensity/ Speed	Distance	Target Heart Rate	Actual Heart Rate	Cal. Burned

Exercise

		Set 1	Set 2	Set 3	Set 4	Set 5	Set 6
	Reps						
	Weight						

How Did The Workout Go ?

Bad Ok Good Great

Date : / / S M T W Th F S

Today I Am Grateful For:

◇

◇

◇

Breakfast

Lunch

Dinner

Snacks

How I Feel Today About My Food :

Water :

Sleep Time :

Cravings / Response

Something To Make Tomorrow Better:

Victory Of The Day:

Notes

Date : / /   S M T W Th F S   Weight   Start

Muscle Group   Stretch ☐ Warm-up ☐   Finish

Affirmation

Cardio

Type	Time	Intensity/ Speed	Distance	Target Heart Rate	Actual Heart Rate	Cal. Burned

Exercise		Set 1	Set 2	Set 3	Set 4	Set 5	Set 6
	Reps						
	Weight						

How Did The Workout Go ?

Bad   Ok   Good   Great

Date : / /

S M T W Th F S

Today I Am Grateful For:

◇

◇

◇

Breakfast

Lunch

Dinner

Snacks

How I Feel Today About My Food :

Water :

Sleep Time :

Cravings / Response

Something To Make Tomorrow Better:

Victory Of The Day:

Notes

Date : / / ☐ ☐ ☐ ☐ ☐ ☐ ☐ Weight Start
S M T W Th F S

Muscle Group Stretch ☐ Warm-up ☐ Finish

Affirmation

Cardio

Type	Time	Intensity/ Speed	Distance	Target Heart Rate	Actual Heart Rate	Cal. Burned

Exercise		Set 1	Set 2	Set 3	Set 4	Set 5	Set 6
	Reps						
	Weight						

How Did The Workout Go ?

Bad Ok Good Great

Date : / /

S M T W Th F S

Today I Am Grateful For:

◇

◇

◇

Breakfast

Lunch

Dinner

Snacks

How I Feel Today About My Food :

Water :

Sleep Time :

Cravings / Response

Something To Make Tomorrow Better:

Victory Of The Day:

Notes

Date : / /

S M T W Th F S

Weight

Start

Muscle Group

Stretch ☐ Warm-up ☐

Finish

Affirmation

Cardio

Type	Time	Intensity/ Speed	Distance	Target Heart Rate	Actual Heart Rate	Cal. Burned

Exercise		Set 1	Set 2	Set 3	Set 4	Set 5	Set 6
	Reps						
	Weight						

How Did The Workout Go ?

Bad Ok Good Great

Date : / /

S M T W Th F S

Today I Am Grateful For:

◇

◇

◇

Breakfast

Lunch

Dinner

Snacks

How I Feel Today About My Food :

Water :

Sleep Time :

Cravings / Response

Something To Make Tomorrow Better:

Victory Of The Day:

Notes

Date : / /

S M T W Th F S

Weight

Start

Muscle Group

Stretch ☐ Warm-up ☐

Finish

Affirmation

Cardio

Type	Time	Intensity/ Speed	Distance	Target Heart Rate	Actual Heart Rate	Cal. Burned

Exercise

Exercise		Set 1	Set 2	Set 3	Set 4	Set 5	Set 6
	Reps						
	Weight						

How Did The Workout Go ?

Bad Ok Good Great

Date : / /

S M T W Th F S

Today I Am Grateful For:

Breakfast

Lunch

Dinner

Snacks

How I Feel Today About My Food :

Water :

Sleep Time :

Cravings / Response

Something To Make Tomorrow Better:

Victory Of The Day:

Notes

Date : / /

S M T W Th F S

Weight

Start

Muscle Group

Stretch ☐ Warm-up ☐

Finish

Affirmation

Cardio

Type	Time	Intensity/ Speed	Distance	Target Heart Rate	Actual Heart Rate	Cal. Burned

Exercise		Set 1	Set 2	Set 3	Set 4	Set 5	Set 6
	Reps						
	Weight						

How Did The Workout Go ?

Bad Ok Good Great

Date : / /

S M T W Th F S

Today I Am Grateful For:

◇

◇

◇

Breakfast

Lunch

Dinner

Snacks

How I Feel Today About My Food :

Water :

Sleep Time :

Cravings / Response

Something To Make Tomorrow Better:

Victory Of The Day:

Notes

Date : / / ☐ S ☐ M ☐ T ☐ W ☐ Th ☐ F ☐ S Weight Start

Muscle Group Stretch ☐ Warm-up ☐ Finish

Affirmation

Cardio

Type	Time	Intensity/ Speed	Distance	Target Heart Rate	Actual Heart Rate	Cal. Burned

Exercise		Set 1	Set 2	Set 3	Set 4	Set 5	Set 6
	Reps						
	Weight						

How Did The Workout Go ?

Bad Ok Good Great

Date : / /

S M T W Th F S

Today I Am Grateful For:

◇

◇

◇

Breakfast

Lunch

Dinner

Snacks

How I Feel Today About My Food :

Water :

Sleep Time :

Cravings / Response

Something To Make Tomorrow Better:

Victory Of The Day:

Notes

Date : / /

S M T W Th F S

Weight

Start

Muscle Group

Stretch ☐ Warm-up ☐

Finish

Affirmation

Cardio

Type	Time	Intensity/ Speed	Distance	Target Heart Rate	Actual Heart Rate	Cal. Burned

Exercise

Exercise		Set 1	Set 2	Set 3	Set 4	Set 5	Set 6
	Reps						
	Weight						

How Did The Workout Go ?

Bad Ok Good Great

Date : / /

S M T W Th F S

Today I Am Grateful For:

◇

◇

◇

Breakfast

Lunch

Dinner

Snacks

How I Feel Today About My Food :

Water :

Sleep Time :

Cravings / Response

Something To Make Tomorrow Better:

Victory Of The Day:

Notes

Date : / /

S M T W Th F S

Weight

Start

Muscle Group

Stretch ☐ Warm-up ☐

Finish

Affirmation

Cardio

Type	Time	Intensity/ Speed	Distance	Target Heart Rate	Actual Heart Rate	Cal. Burned

Exercise

Exercise		Set 1	Set 2	Set 3	Set 4	Set 5	Set 6
	Reps						
	Weight						

How Did The Workout Go ?

Bad Ok Good Great

Date : / /

S M T W Th F S

Today I Am Grateful For:

◇

◇

◇

Breakfast

Lunch

Dinner

Snacks

How I Feel Today About My Food :

Water :

Sleep Time :

Cravings / Response

Something To Make Tomorrow Better:

Victory Of The Day:

Notes

Date : / /

☐ S ☐ M ☐ T ☐ W ☐ Th ☐ F ☐ S

Weight

Start

Muscle Group

Stretch ☐ Warm-up ☐

Finish

Affirmation

Cardio

Type	Time	Intensity/ Speed	Distance	Target Heart Rate	Actual Heart Rate	Cal. Burned

Exercise		Set 1	Set 2	Set 3	Set 4	Set 5	Set 6
	Reps						
	Weight						

How Did The Workout Go ?

☐ Bad ☐ Ok ☐ Good ☐ Great

Date : / /

S M T W Th F S

Today I Am Grateful For:

◇

◇

◇

Breakfast

Lunch

Dinner

Snacks

How I Feel Today About My Food :

Water :

Sleep Time :

Cravings / Response

Something To Make Tomorrow Better:

Victory Of The Day:

Notes

Date : / / ☐ ☐ ☐ ☐ ☐ ☐ ☐ S M T W Th F S Weight Start

Muscle Group Stretch ☐ Warm-up ☐ Finish

Affirmation

Cardio

Type	Time	Intensity/ Speed	Distance	Target Heart Rate	Actual Heart Rate	Cal. Burned

Exercise

Exercise		Set 1	Set 2	Set 3	Set 4	Set 5	Set 6
	Reps						
	Weight						

How Did The Workout Go ?

Bad Ok Good Great

Date : / /

S M T W Th F S

Today I Am Grateful For:

◇

◇

◇

Breakfast

Lunch

Dinner

Snacks

How I Feel Today About My Food :

Water :

Sleep Time :

Cravings / Response

Something To Make Tomorrow Better:

Victory Of The Day:

Notes

Date : / /

S M T W Th F S

Weight

Start

Muscle Group

Stretch ☐ Warm-up ☐

Finish

Affirmation

Cardio

Type	Time	Intensity/ Speed	Distance	Target Heart Rate	Actual Heart Rate	Cal. Burned

Exercise		Set 1	Set 2	Set 3	Set 4	Set 5	Set 6
	Reps						
	Weight						

How Did The Workout Go ?

Bad Ok Good Great

Date : / /

S M T W Th F S

Today I Am Grateful For:

Breakfast

Lunch

Dinner

Snacks

How I Feel Today About My Food :

Water :

Sleep Time :

Cravings / Response

Something To Make Tomorrow Better:

Victory Of The Day:

Notes

Date : / /

S M T W Th F S

Weight

Start

Muscle Group

Stretch ☐ Warm-up ☐

Finish

Affirmation

Cardio

Type	Time	Intensity/ Speed	Distance	Target Heart Rate	Actual Heart Rate	Cal. Burned

Exercise		Set 1	Set 2	Set 3	Set 4	Set 5	Set 6
	Reps						
	Weight						

How Did The Workout Go ?

Bad Ok Good Great

Date : / /

S M T W Th F S

Today I Am Grateful For:

◇

◇

◇

Breakfast

Lunch

Dinner

Snacks

How I Feel Today About My Food :

Water :

Sleep Time :

Cravings / Response

Something To Make Tomorrow Better:

Victory Of The Day:

Notes

Date : / /

S M T W Th F S

Weight

Start

Muscle Group

Stretch ☐ Warm-up ☐

Finish

Affirmation

Cardio

Type	Time	Intensity/ Speed	Distance	Target Heart Rate	Actual Heart Rate	Cal. Burned

Exercise		Set 1	Set 2	Set 3	Set 4	Set 5	Set 6
	Reps						
	Weight						

How Did The Workout Go ?

Bad Ok Good Great

Date :   /   /

S M T W Th F S

Today I Am Grateful For:

◇

◇

◇

Breakfast

Lunch

Dinner

Snacks

How I Feel Today About My Food :

Water :

Sleep Time :

Cravings / Response

Something To Make Tomorrow Better:

Victory Of The Day:

Notes

Date : / /

☐ S ☐ M ☐ T ☐ W ☐ Th ☐ F ☐ S

Weight

Start

Muscle Group

Stretch ☐ Warm-up ☐

Finish

Affirmation

Cardio

Type	Time	Intensity/ Speed	Distance	Target Heart Rate	Actual Heart Rate	Cal. Burned

Exercise

Exercise		Set 1	Set 2	Set 3	Set 4	Set 5	Set 6
	Reps						
	Weight						

How Did The Workout Go ?

Bad Ok Good Great

Date : / / S M T W Th F S

Today I Am Grateful For:

◇

◇

◇

Breakfast

Lunch

Dinner

Snacks

How I Feel Today About My Food :

Water :

Sleep Time :

Cravings / Response

Something To Make Tomorrow Better:

Victory Of The Day:

Notes

Date : / / ☐ ☐ ☐ ☐ ☐ ☐ ☐ S M T W Th F S Weight Start

Muscle Group Stretch ☐ Warm-up ☐ Finish

Affirmation

Cardio

Type	Time	Intensity/ Speed	Distance	Target Heart Rate	Actual Heart Rate	Cal. Burned

Exercise		Set 1	Set 2	Set 3	Set 4	Set 5	Set 6
	Reps						
	Weight						

How Did The Workout Go ?

Bad | Ok | Good | Great

Date : / /

S M T W Th F S

Today I Am Grateful For:

◇

◇

◇

Breakfast

Lunch

Dinner

Snacks

How I Feel Today About My Food :

Water :

Sleep Time :

Cravings / Response

Something To Make Tomorrow Better:

Victory Of The Day:

Notes

Date : / /

S M T W Th F S

Weight

Start

Muscle Group

Stretch ☐ Warm-up ☐

Finish

Affirmation

Cardio

Type	Time	Intensity/ Speed	Distance	Target Heart Rate	Actual Heart Rate	Cal. Burned

Exercise		Set 1	Set 2	Set 3	Set 4	Set 5	Set 6
	Reps						
	Weight						

How Did The Workout Go ?

Bad Ok Good Great

Date : / /

S M T W Th F S

Today I Am Grateful For:

◇

◇

◇

Breakfast

Lunch

Dinner

Snacks

How I Feel Today About My Food :

Water :

Sleep Time :

Cravings / Response

Something To Make Tomorrow Better:

Victory Of The Day:

Notes

Date : / / ☐ ☐ ☐ ☐ ☐ ☐ ☐ Weight Start

S M T W Th F S

Muscle Group Stretch ☐ Warm-up ☐ Finish

Affirmation

Cardio

Type	Time	Intensity/ Speed	Distance	Target Heart Rate	Actual Heart Rate	Cal. Burned

Exercise

Exercise		Set 1	Set 2	Set 3	Set 4	Set 5	Set 6
	Reps						
	Weight						

How Did The Workout Go ?

Bad Ok Good Great

Date : / / S M T W Th F S

Today I Am Grateful For:

◇

◇

◇

Breakfast

Lunch

Dinner

Snacks

How I Feel Today About My Food :

Water :

Sleep Time :

Cravings / Response

Something To Make Tomorrow Better:

Victory Of The Day:

Notes

Date : / /

S M T W Th F S

Weight

Start

Muscle Group

Stretch ☐ Warm-up ☐

Finish

Affirmation

Cardio

Type	Time	Intensity/ Speed	Distance	Target Heart Rate	Actual Heart Rate	Cal. Burned

Exercise

		Set 1	Set 2	Set 3	Set 4	Set 5	Set 6
	Reps						
	Weight						

How Did The Workout Go ?

Bad Ok Good Great

Date : / /

S M T W Th F S

Today I Am Grateful For:

◇

◇

◇

Breakfast

Lunch

Dinner

Snacks

How I Feel Today About My Food :

Water :

Sleep Time :

Cravings / Response

Something To Make Tomorrow Better:

Victory Of The Day:

Notes

Date : / /

S M T W Th F S

Weight

Start

Muscle Group

Stretch ☐ Warm-up ☐

Finish

Affirmation

Cardio

Type	Time	Intensity/ Speed	Distance	Target Heart Rate	Actual Heart Rate	Cal. Burned

Exercise		Set 1	Set 2	Set 3	Set 4	Set 5	Set 6
	Reps						
	Weight						

How Did The Workout Go ?

Bad Ok Good Great

Date : / /

S M T W Th F S

Today I Am Grateful For:

◇

◇

◇

Breakfast

Lunch

Dinner

Snacks

How I Feel Today About My Food :

Water :

Sleep Time :

Cravings / Response

Something To Make Tomorrow Better:

Victory Of The Day:

Notes

Date : / /

S M T W Th F S

Weight

Start

Muscle Group

Stretch ☐ Warm-up ☐

Finish

Affirmation

Cardio

Type	Time	Intensity/ Speed	Distance	Target Heart Rate	Actual Heart Rate	Cal. Burned

Exercise		Set 1	Set 2	Set 3	Set 4	Set 5	Set 6
	Reps						
	Weight						

How Did The Workout Go ?

Bad | Ok | Good | Great

Date : / /

S M T W Th F S

How I Feel Today About My Food :

Today I Am Grateful For:

◇

◇

◇

Water :

Sleep Time :

Cravings / Response

Breakfast

Something To Make Tomorrow Better:

Lunch

Victory Of The Day:

Dinner

Notes

Snacks

Date : / / ☐ S ☐ M ☐ T ☐ W ☐ Th ☐ F ☐ S

Weight

Start

Muscle Group

Stretch ☐ Warm-up ☐

Finish

Affirmation

Cardio

Type	Time	Intensity/ Speed	Distance	Target Heart Rate	Actual Heart Rate	Cal. Burned

Exercise

		Set 1	Set 2	Set 3	Set 4	Set 5	Set 6
	Reps						
	Weight						

How Did The Workout Go ?

Bad | Ok | Good | Great

Date : / /

S M T W Th F S

How I Feel Today About My Food :

Today I Am Grateful For:

◇

◇

◇

Water :

Sleep Time :

Cravings / Response

Breakfast

Something To Make Tomorrow Better:

Lunch

Victory Of The Day:

Dinner

Notes

Snacks

Date : / / ☐ ☐ ☐ ☐ ☐ ☐ ☐ Weight Start
S M T W Th F S

Muscle Group Stretch ☐ Warm-up ☐ Finish

Affirmation

Cardio

Type	Time	Intensity/ Speed	Distance	Target Heart Rate	Actual Heart Rate	Cal. Burned

Exercise

Exercise		Set 1	Set 2	Set 3	Set 4	Set 5	Set 6
	Reps						
	Weight						

How Did The Workout Go ?

Bad Ok Good Great

Date : / /

S M T W Th F S

Today I Am Grateful For:

◇

◇

◇

Breakfast

Lunch

Dinner

Snacks

How I Feel Today About My Food :

Water :

Sleep Time :

Cravings / Response

Something To Make Tomorrow Better:

Victory Of The Day:

Notes

Date : / / S M T W Th F S Weight Start

Muscle Group Stretch ☐ Warm-up ☐ Finish

Affirmation

Cardio

Type	Time	Intensity/ Speed	Distance	Target Heart Rate	Actual Heart Rate	Cal. Burned

Exercise		Set 1	Set 2	Set 3	Set 4	Set 5	Set 6
	Reps						
	Weight						

How Did The Workout Go ?

Bad Ok Good Great

Date : / /

S M T W Th F S

Today I Am Grateful For:

◇

◇

◇

Breakfast

Lunch

Dinner

Snacks

How I Feel Today About My Food :

Water :

Sleep Time :

Cravings / Response

Something To Make Tomorrow Better:

Victory Of The Day:

Notes

Date : / / S M T W Th F S Weight Start

Muscle Group Stretch ☐ Warm-up ☐ Finish

Affirmation

Cardio

Type	Time	Intensity/ Speed	Distance	Target Heart Rate	Actual Heart Rate	Cal. Burned

Exercise

Exercise		Set 1	Set 2	Set 3	Set 4	Set 5	Set 6
	Reps						
	Weight						

How Did The Workout Go ?

Bad Ok Good Great

Date : / / S M T W Th F S

Today I Am Grateful For:

◇

◇

◇

Breakfast

Lunch

Dinner

Snacks

How I Feel Today About My Food :

Water :

Sleep Time :

Cravings / Response

Something To Make Tomorrow Better:

Victory Of The Day:

Notes

Date : / / ☐ ☐ ☐ ☐ ☐ ☐ ☐ S M T W Th F S Weight Start

Muscle Group Stretch ☐ Warm-up ☐ Finish

Affirmation

Cardio

Type	Time	Intensity/ Speed	Distance	Target Heart Rate	Actual Heart Rate	Cal. Burned

Exercise

Exercise		Set 1	Set 2	Set 3	Set 4	Set 5	Set 6
	Reps						
	Weight						

How Did The Workout Go ?

Bad Ok Good Great

Results

Date : / /

Weight

Body Fat %

Height

Front Image

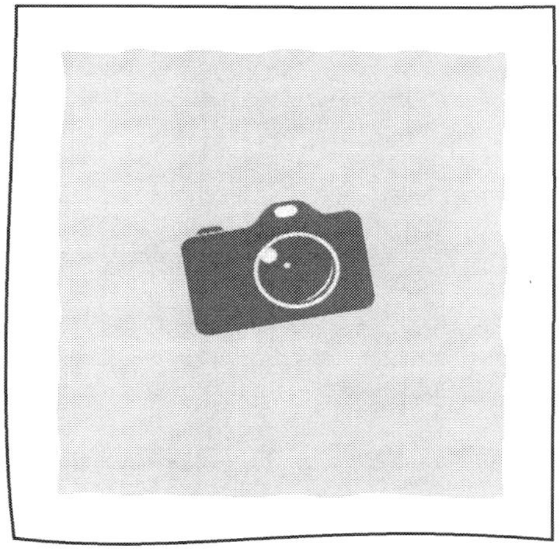

Side Image

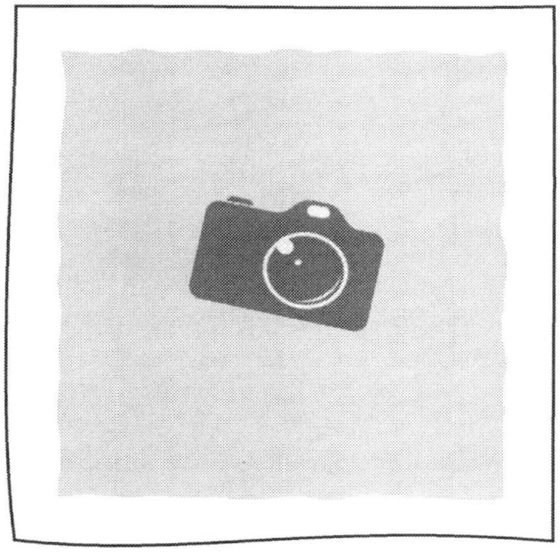

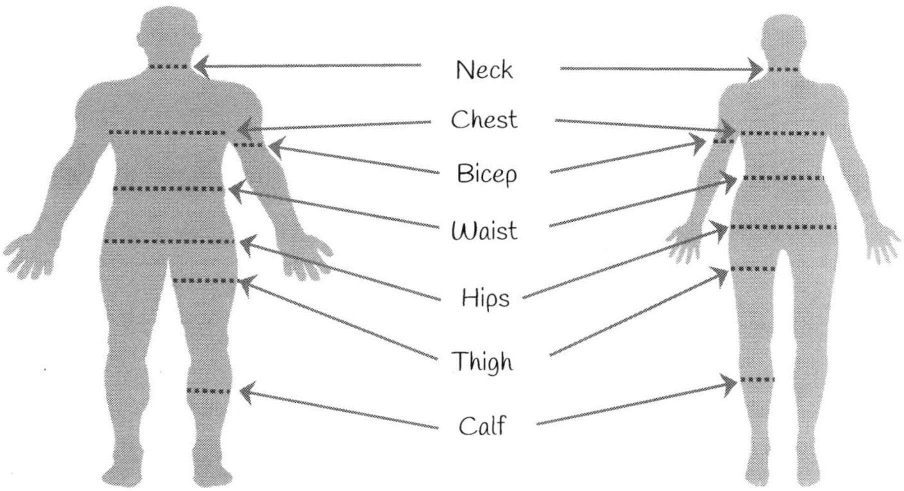

Measurements

Neck

Chest

Bicep

Waist

Hips

Thigh

Calf

My Goals

Goal #1

Plan

Deadline

Reward If Achieved

Goal #2

Plan

Deadline

Reward If Achieved

Goal #3

Plan

Deadline

Reward If Achieved

Goal #4

Plan

Deadline

Reward If Achieved

Goal #5

Plan

Deadline

Reward If Achieved

Notes

Date : / / S M T W Th F S

Today I Am Grateful For:

◇

◇

◇

Breakfast

Lunch

Dinner

Snacks

How I Feel Today About My Food :

Water :

Sleep Time :

Cravings / Response

Something To Make Tomorrow Better:

Victory Of The Day:

Notes

Date : / / ☐ S ☐ M ☐ T ☐ W ☐ Th ☐ F ☐ S Weight Start

Muscle Group Stretch ☐ Warm-up ☐ Finish

Affirmation

Cardio

Type	Time	Intensity/ Speed	Distance	Target Heart Rate	Actual Heart Rate	Cal. Burned

Exercise

Exercise		Set 1	Set 2	Set 3	Set 4	Set 5	Set 6
	Reps						
	Weight						

How Did The Workout Go ?

Bad Ok Good Great

Date : / /

S M T W Th F S

Today I Am Grateful For:

◇

◇

◇

Breakfast

Lunch

Dinner

Snacks

How I Feel Today About My Food :

Water :

Sleep Time :

Cravings / Response

Something To Make Tomorrow Better:

Victory Of The Day:

Notes

Date : / / ☐ ☐ ☐ ☐ ☐ ☐ ☐ Weight Start
S M T W Th F S

Muscle Group Stretch ☐ Warm-up ☐ Finish

Affirmation

Cardio

Type	Time	Intensity/ Speed	Distance	Target Heart Rate	Actual Heart Rate	Cal. Burned

Exercise

Exercise		Set 1	Set 2	Set 3	Set 4	Set 5	Set 6
	Reps						
	Weight						

How Did The Workout Go ?

Bad | Ok | Good | Great

Date : / /

S M T W Th F S

Today I Am Grateful For:

◇

◇

◇

Breakfast

Lunch

Dinner

Snacks

How I Feel Today About My Food :

Water :

Sleep Time :

Cravings / Response

Something To Make Tomorrow Better:

Victory Of The Day:

Notes

Date : / /

S M T W Th F S

Weight

Start

Muscle Group

Stretch ☐ Warm-up ☐

Finish

Affirmation

Cardio

Type	Time	Intensity/ Speed	Distance	Target Heart Rate	Actual Heart Rate	Cal. Burned

Exercise		Set 1	Set 2	Set 3	Set 4	Set 5	Set 6
	Reps						
	Weight						

How Did The Workout Go ?

Bad Ok Good Great

Date : / /

S M T W Th F S

Today I Am Grateful For:

◇

◇

◇

Breakfast

Lunch

Dinner

Snacks

How I Feel Today About My Food :

Water :

Sleep Time :

Cravings / Response

Something To Make Tomorrow Better:

Victory Of The Day:

Notes

Date : / / ☐ ☐ ☐ ☐ ☐ ☐ ☐ S M T W Th F S Weight Start

Muscle Group Stretch ☐ Warm-up ☐ Finish

Affirmation

Cardio

Type	Time	Intensity/ Speed	Distance	Target Heart Rate	Actual Heart Rate	Cal. Burned

Exercise

Exercise		Set 1	Set 2	Set 3	Set 4	Set 5	Set 6
	Reps						
	Weight						

How Did The Workout Go ?

Bad Ok Good Great

Date : / / S M T W Th F S

Today I Am Grateful For:

◇

◇

◇

Breakfast

Lunch

Dinner

Snacks

How I Feel Today About My Food :

Water :

Sleep Time :

Cravings / Response

Something To Make Tomorrow Better:

Victory Of The Day:

Notes

Date : / /

S M T W Th F S

Weight

Start

Muscle Group

Stretch ☐ Warm-up ☐

Finish

Affirmation

Cardio

Type	Time	Intensity/ Speed	Distance	Target Heart Rate	Actual Heart Rate	Cal. Burned

Exercise

Exercise		Set 1	Set 2	Set 3	Set 4	Set 5	Set 6
	Reps						
	Weight						

How Did The Workout Go ?

Bad Ok Good Great

Date : / /

S M T W Th F S

Today I Am Grateful For:

◇

◇

◇

Breakfast

Lunch

Dinner

Snacks

How I Feel Today About My Food :

Water :

Sleep Time :

Cravings / Response

Something To Make Tomorrow Better:

Victory Of The Day:

Notes

Date : / /

S M T W Th F S

Weight

Start

Muscle Group

Stretch ☐ Warm-up ☐

Finish

Affirmation

Cardio

Type	Time	Intensity/ Speed	Distance	Target Heart Rate	Actual Heart Rate	Cal. Burned

Exercise

Exercise		Set 1	Set 2	Set 3	Set 4	Set 5	Set 6
	Reps						
	Weight						

How Did The Workout Go ?

Bad Ok Good Great

Date : / / S M T W Th F S

Today I Am Grateful For:

◇

◇

◇

Breakfast

Lunch

Dinner

Snacks

How I Feel Today About My Food :

Water :

Sleep Time :

Cravings / Response

Something To Make Tomorrow Better:

Victory Of The Day:

Notes

Date : / /

S M T W Th F S

Weight

Start

Muscle Group

Stretch ☐ Warm-up ☐

Finish

Affirmation

Cardio

Type	Time	Intensity/ Speed	Distance	Target Heart Rate	Actual Heart Rate	Cal. Burned

Exercise		Set 1	Set 2	Set 3	Set 4	Set 5	Set 6
	Reps						
	Weight						

How Did The Workout Go ?

Bad Ok Good Great

Date : / /

S M T W Th F S

Today I Am Grateful For:

◇

◇

◇

Breakfast

Lunch

Dinner

Snacks

How I Feel Today About My Food :

Water :

Sleep Time :

Cravings / Response

Something To Make Tomorrow Better:

Victory Of The Day:

Notes

Date : / /　☐ S ☐ M ☐ T ☐ W ☐ Th ☐ F ☐ S　Weight　Start

Muscle Group　Stretch ☐ Warm-up ☐　Finish

Affirmation

Cardio

Type	Time	Intensity/ Speed	Distance	Target Heart Rate	Actual Heart Rate	Cal. Burned

Exercise		Set 1	Set 2	Set 3	Set 4	Set 5	Set 6
	Reps						
	Weight						

How Did The Workout Go ?

☐ Bad　☐ Ok　☐ Good　☐ Great

Date : / /

S M T W Th F S

Today I Am Grateful For:

◇

◇

◇

Breakfast

Lunch

Dinner

Snacks

How I Feel Today About My Food :

Water :

Sleep Time :

Cravings / Response

Something To Make Tomorrow Better:

Victory Of The Day:

Notes

Date : / / ☐ ☐ ☐ ☐ ☐ ☐ ☐ Weight Start

S M T W Th F S

Muscle Group Stretch ☐ Warm-up ☐ Finish

Affirmation

Cardio

Type	Time	Intensity/ Speed	Distance	Target Heart Rate	Actual Heart Rate	Cal. Burned

Exercise		Set 1	Set 2	Set 3	Set 4	Set 5	Set 6
	Reps						
	Weight						

How Did The Workout Go ?

Bad Ok Good Great

Date : / /

S M T W Th F S

Today I Am Grateful For:

◇

◇

◇

Breakfast

Lunch

Dinner

Snacks

How I Feel Today About My Food :

Water :

Sleep Time :

Cravings / Response

Something To Make Tomorrow Better:

Victory Of The Day:

Notes

Date : / / ☐☐☐☐☐☐☐ S M T W Th F S Weight Start

Muscle Group Stretch ☐ Warm-up ☐ Finish

Affirmation

Cardio

Type	Time	Intensity/ Speed	Distance	Target Heart Rate	Actual Heart Rate	Cal. Burned

Exercise		Set 1	Set 2	Set 3	Set 4	Set 5	Set 6
	Reps						
	Weight						

How Did The Workout Go ?

Bad Ok Good Great

Date : / / S M T W Th F S

Today I Am Grateful For:

◇

◇

◇

Breakfast

Lunch

Dinner

Snacks

How I Feel Today About My Food :

Water :

Sleep Time :

Cravings / Response

Something To Make Tomorrow Better:

Victory Of The Day:

Notes

Date : / / ☐ ☐ ☐ ☐ ☐ ☐ ☐ S M T W Th F S Weight Start

Muscle Group Stretch ☐ Warm-up ☐ Finish

Affirmation

Cardio

Type	Time	Intensity/ Speed	Distance	Target Heart Rate	Actual Heart Rate	Cal. Burned

Exercise

Exercise		Set 1	Set 2	Set 3	Set 4	Set 5	Set 6
	Reps						
	Weight						

How Did The Workout Go ?

Bad Ok Good Great

Date : / / S M T W Th F S

How I Feel Today About My Food :

Today I Am Grateful For:

◇

◇

◇

Water :

Sleep Time :

Breakfast

Cravings / Response

Lunch

Something To Make Tomorrow Better:

Dinner

Victory Of The Day:

Snacks

Notes

Date : / /

S M T W Th F S

Weight

Start

Muscle Group

Stretch ☐ Warm-up ☐

Finish

Affirmation

Cardio

Type	Time	Intensity/ Speed	Distance	Target Heart Rate	Actual Heart Rate	Cal. Burned

Exercise

Exercise		Set 1	Set 2	Set 3	Set 4	Set 5	Set 6
	Reps						
	Weight						

How Did The Workout Go ?

Bad Ok Good Great

Date : / /

S M T W Th F S

Today I Am Grateful For:

◇

◇

◇

Breakfast

Lunch

Dinner

Snacks

How I Feel Today About My Food :

Water :

Sleep Time :

Cravings / Response

Something To Make Tomorrow Better:

Victory Of The Day:

Notes

Date : / / ☐ ☐ ☐ ☐ ☐ ☐ ☐ Weight Start
S M T W Th F S

Muscle Group Stretch ☐ Warm-up ☐ Finish

Affirmation

Cardio

Type	Time	Intensity/ Speed	Distance	Target Heart Rate	Actual Heart Rate	Cal. Burned

Exercise

Exercise		Set 1	Set 2	Set 3	Set 4	Set 5	Set 6
	Reps						
	Weight						

How Did The Workout Go ?

Bad Ok Good Great

Date : / /

S M T W Th F S

Today I Am Grateful For:

◇

◇

◇

Breakfast

Lunch

Dinner

Snacks

How I Feel Today About My Food :

Water :

Sleep Time :

Cravings / Response

Something To Make Tomorrow Better:

Victory Of The Day:

Notes

Date : / / ☐ ☐ ☐ ☐ ☐ ☐ ☐ Weight Start

S M T W Th F S

Muscle Group Stretch ☐ Warm-up ☐ Finish

Affirmation

Cardio

Type	Time	Intensity/ Speed	Distance	Target Heart Rate	Actual Heart Rate	Cal. Burned

Exercise		Set 1	Set 2	Set 3	Set 4	Set 5	Set 6
	Reps						
	Weight						

How Did The Workout Go ?

Bad Ok Good Great

Date : / / S M T W Th F S

How I Feel Today About My Food :

Today I Am Grateful For:

◇

◇

◇

Water :

Sleep Time :

Cravings / Response

Breakfast

Something To Make Tomorrow Better:

Lunch

Victory Of The Day:

Dinner

Notes

Snacks

Date : / /

S M T W Th F S

Weight

Start

Muscle Group

Stretch ☐ Warm-up ☐

Finish

Affirmation

Cardio

Type	Time	Intensity/ Speed	Distance	Target Heart Rate	Actual Heart Rate	Cal. Burned

Exercise		Set 1	Set 2	Set 3	Set 4	Set 5	Set 6
	Reps						
	Weight						

How Did The Workout Go ?

Bad Ok Good Great

Date : / /

S M T W Th F S

Today I Am Grateful For:

Breakfast

Lunch

Dinner

Snacks

How I Feel Today About My Food :

Water :

Sleep Time :

Cravings / Response

Something To Make Tomorrow Better:

Victory Of The Day:

Notes

Date : / / ☐ ☐ ☐ ☐ ☐ ☐ ☐ S M T W Th F S Weight Start

Muscle Group Stretch ☐ Warm-up ☐ Finish

Affirmation

Cardio

Type	Time	Intensity/ Speed	Distance	Target Heart Rate	Actual Heart Rate	Cal. Burned

Exercise

Exercise		Set 1	Set 2	Set 3	Set 4	Set 5	Set 6
	Reps						
	Weight						

How Did The Workout Go ?

Bad Ok Good Great

Date : / / S M T W Th F S

Today I Am Grateful For:

◇

◇

◇

Breakfast

Lunch

Dinner

Snacks

How I Feel Today About My Food :

Water :

Sleep Time :

Cravings / Response

Something To Make Tomorrow Better:

Victory Of The Day:

Notes

Date : / / S M T W Th F S

Weight

Start

Muscle Group

Stretch ☐ Warm-up ☐

Finish

Affirmation

Cardio

Type	Time	Intensity/ Speed	Distance	Target Heart Rate	Actual Heart Rate	Cal. Burned

Exercise		Set 1	Set 2	Set 3	Set 4	Set 5	Set 6
	Reps						
	Weight						

How Did The Workout Go ?

Bad Ok Good Great

Date : / /

S M T W Th F S

Today I Am Grateful For:

◇

◇

◇

Breakfast

Lunch

Dinner

Snacks

How I Feel Today About My Food :

Water :

Sleep Time :

Cravings / Response

Something To Make Tomorrow Better:

Victory Of The Day:

Notes

Date : / / S M T W Th F S Weight Start

Muscle Group Stretch Warm-up Finish

Affirmation

Cardio

Type	Time	Intensity/ Speed	Distance	Target Heart Rate	Actual Heart Rate	Cal. Burned

Exercise		Set 1	Set 2	Set 3	Set 4	Set 5	Set 6
	Reps						
	Weight						

How Did The Workout Go ?

Bad Ok Good Great

Date : / /

S M T W Th F S

Today I Am Grateful For:

◇

◇

◇

Breakfast

Lunch

Dinner

Snacks

How I Feel Today About My Food :

Water :

Sleep Time :

Cravings / Response

Something To Make Tomorrow Better:

Victory Of The Day:

Notes

Date : / /

S M T W Th F S

Weight

Start

Muscle Group

Stretch ☐ Warm-up ☐

Finish

Affirmation

Cardio

Type	Time	Intensity/ Speed	Distance	Target Heart Rate	Actual Heart Rate	Cal. Burned

Exercise

Exercise		Set 1	Set 2	Set 3	Set 4	Set 5	Set 6
	Reps						
	Weight						

How Did The Workout Go ?

Bad Ok Good Great

Date : / /

S M T W Th F S

Today I Am Grateful For:

Breakfast

Lunch

Dinner

Snacks

How I Feel Today About My Food :

Water :

Sleep Time :

Cravings / Response

Something To Make Tomorrow Better:

Victory Of The Day:

Notes

Date : / /

S M T W Th F S

Weight

Start

Muscle Group

Stretch ☐ Warm-up ☐

Finish

Affirmation

Cardio

Type	Time	Intensity/ Speed	Distance	Target Heart Rate	Actual Heart Rate	Cal. Burned

Exercise

Exercise		Set 1	Set 2	Set 3	Set 4	Set 5	Set 6
	Reps						
	Weight						

How Did The Workout Go ?

Bad Ok Good Great

Date : / /

S M T W Th F S

Today I Am Grateful For:

◇

◇

◇

Breakfast

Lunch

Dinner

Snacks

How I Feel Today About My Food :

Water :

Sleep Time :

Cravings / Response

Something To Make Tomorrow Better:

Victory Of The Day:

Notes

Date : / /

S M T W Th F S

Weight Start

Muscle Group

Stretch ☐ Warm-up ☐ Finish

Affirmation

Cardio

Type	Time	Intensity/ Speed	Distance	Target Heart Rate	Actual Heart Rate	Cal. Burned

Exercise

Exercise		Set 1	Set 2	Set 3	Set 4	Set 5	Set 6
	Reps						
	Weight						

How Did The Workout Go ?

Bad Ok Good Great

Date : / /

S M T W Th F S

Today I Am Grateful For:

◇

◇

◇

Breakfast

Lunch

Dinner

Snacks

How I Feel Today About My Food :

Water :

Sleep Time :

Cravings / Response

Something To Make Tomorrow Better:

Victory Of The Day:

Notes

Date : / / ☐ ☐ ☐ ☐ ☐ ☐ ☐ S M T W Th F S

Weight

Start

Muscle Group

Stretch ☐ Warm-up ☐

Finish

Affirmation

Cardio

Type	Time	Intensity/ Speed	Distance	Target Heart Rate	Actual Heart Rate	Cal. Burned

Exercise		Set 1	Set 2	Set 3	Set 4	Set 5	Set 6
	Reps						
	Weight						

How Did The Workout Go ?

Bad | Ok | Good | Great

Date : / /

S M T W Th F S

How I Feel Today About My Food :

Water :

Sleep Time :

Today I Am Grateful For:

◇

◇

◇

Breakfast

Lunch

Dinner

Snacks

Cravings / Response

Something To Make Tomorrow Better:

Victory Of The Day:

Notes

Date : / / ☐ ☐ ☐ ☐ ☐ ☐ ☐ S M T W Th F S Weight Start

Muscle Group Stretch ☐ Warm-up ☐ Finish

Affirmation

Cardio

Type	Time	Intensity/ Speed	Distance	Target Heart Rate	Actual Heart Rate	Cal. Burned

Exercise

Exercise		Set 1	Set 2	Set 3	Set 4	Set 5	Set 6
	Reps						
	Weight						

How Did The Workout Go ?

Bad Ok Good Great

Date : / / S M T W Th F S

Today I Am Grateful For:

◇

◇

◇

Breakfast

Lunch

Dinner

Snacks

How I Feel Today About My Food :

Water :

Sleep Time :

Cravings / Response

Something To Make Tomorrow Better:

Victory Of The Day:

Notes

Date : / / S M T W Th F S

Weight Start

Muscle Group

Stretch ☐ Warm-up ☐ Finish

Affirmation

Cardio

Type	Time	Intensity/ Speed	Distance	Target Heart Rate	Actual Heart Rate	Cal. Burned

Exercise		Set 1	Set 2	Set 3	Set 4	Set 5	Set 6
	Reps						
	Weight						

How Did The Workout Go ?

Bad Ok Good Great

Date : / /

S M T W Th F S

Today I Am Grateful For:

Breakfast

Lunch

Dinner

Snacks

How I Feel Today About My Food :

Water :

Sleep Time :

Cravings / Response

Something To Make Tomorrow Better:

Victory Of The Day:

Notes

Date : / / S M T W Th F S Weight Start

Muscle Group Stretch ☐ Warm-up ☐ Finish

Affirmation

Cardio

Type	Time	Intensity/ Speed	Distance	Target Heart Rate	Actual Heart Rate	Cal. Burned

Exercise

		Set 1	Set 2	Set 3	Set 4	Set 5	Set 6
	Reps						
	Weight						

How Did The Workout Go ?

Bad Ok Good Great

Date : / /

S M T W Th F S

Today I Am Grateful For:

◇

◇

◇

Breakfast

Lunch

Dinner

Snacks

How I Feel Today About My Food :

Water :

Sleep Time :

Cravings / Response

Something To Make Tomorrow Better:

Victory Of The Day:

Notes

Date : / / ☐ ☐ ☐ ☐ ☐ ☐ ☐ S M T W Th F S Weight Start

Muscle Group Stretch ☐ Warm-up ☐ Finish

Affirmation

Cardio

Type	Time	Intensity/ Speed	Distance	Target Heart Rate	Actual Heart Rate	Cal. Burned

Exercise

		Set 1	Set 2	Set 3	Set 4	Set 5	Set 6
	Reps						
	Weight						

How Did The Workout Go ?

☐ Bad ☐ Ok ☐ Good ☐ Great

Date : / /

S M T W Th F S

Today I Am Grateful For:

Breakfast

Lunch

Dinner

Snacks

How I Feel Today About My Food :

Water :

Sleep Time :

Cravings / Response

Something To Make Tomorrow Better:

Victory Of The Day:

Notes

Date : / /

S M T W Th F S

Weight

Start

Muscle Group

Stretch ☐ Warm-up ☐

Finish

Affirmation

Cardio

Type	Time	Intensity/ Speed	Distance	Target Heart Rate	Actual Heart Rate	Cal. Burned

Exercise

Exercise		Set 1	Set 2	Set 3	Set 4	Set 5	Set 6
	Reps						
	Weight						

How Did The Workout Go ?

Bad | Ok | Good | Great

Date : / / S M T W Th F S

Today I Am Grateful For:

◇

◇

◇

Breakfast

Lunch

Dinner

Snacks

How I Feel Today About My Food :

Water :

Sleep Time :

Cravings / Response

Something To Make Tomorrow Better:

Victory Of The Day:

Notes

Date : / /

S	M	T	W	Th	F	S
☐	☐	☐	☐	☐	☐	☐

Weight

Start

Muscle Group

Stretch ☐ Warm-up ☐

Finish

Affirmation

Cardio

Type	Time	Intensity/ Speed	Distance	Target Heart Rate	Actual Heart Rate	Cal. Burned

Exercise

Exercise		Set 1	Set 2	Set 3	Set 4	Set 5	Set 6
	Reps						
	Weight						

How Did The Workout Go ?

Bad Ok Good Great

Date : / / S M T W Th F S

How I Feel Today About My Food :

Today I Am Grateful For:

◇

◇

◇

Water :

Sleep Time :

Cravings / Response

Breakfast

Something To Make Tomorrow Better:

Lunch

Victory Of The Day:

Dinner

Notes

Snacks

Date : / /

☐ ☐ ☐ ☐ ☐ ☐ ☐
S M T W Th F S

Weight

Start

Muscle Group

Stretch ☐ Warm-up ☐

Finish

Affirmation

Cardio

Type	Time	Intensity/ Speed	Distance	Target Heart Rate	Actual Heart Rate	Cal. Burned

Exercise

Exercise		Set 1	Set 2	Set 3	Set 4	Set 5	Set 6
	Reps						
	Weight						

How Did The Workout Go ?

Bad | Ok | Good | Great

Date : / /

S M T W Th F S

How I Feel Today About My Food :

Today I Am Grateful For:

◇

◇

◇

Water :

Sleep Time :

Cravings / Response

Breakfast

Something To Make Tomorrow Better:

Lunch

Victory Of The Day:

Dinner

Notes

Snacks

Date : / / ☐ ☐ ☐ ☐ ☐ ☐ ☐ Weight Start
S M T W Th F S

Muscle Group Stretch ☐ Warm-up ☐ Finish

Affirmation

Cardio

Type	Time	Intensity/ Speed	Distance	Target Heart Rate	Actual Heart Rate	Cal. Burned

Exercise		Set 1	Set 2	Set 3	Set 4	Set 5	Set 6
	Reps						
	Weight						

How Did The Workout Go ?

Bad Ok Good Great

Results

Date : / /

Weight

Body Fat %

Height

Front Image

Side Image

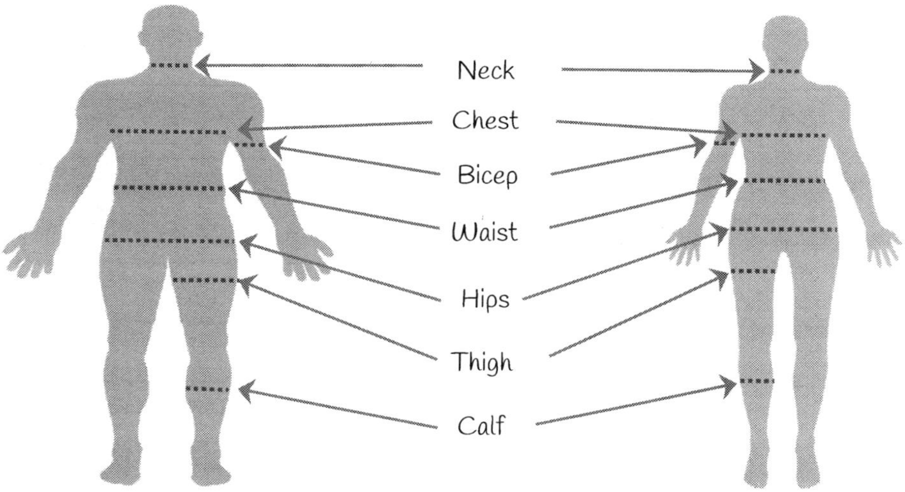

Measurements

Neck

Chest

Bicep

Waist

Hips

Thigh

Calf

Notes

Made in United States
Troutdale, OR
11/03/2026

56847368R00108